Miracle Powder for Quick Weight Loss

Herbal Remedies for Natural Weight Loss and Burns Belly Fat Quickly

Dan Phillips PhD

~DEDICATION~

~LARRY~

For your unwavering support, encouragement, and friendship. Your presence in my life has been a constant source of inspiration. Thank you for your invaluable kindness and belief in my journey. This book is a token of appreciation for your enduring friendship and steadfast encouragement.

TABLE OF CONTENT

CHAPTER 1

Introduction to the Miracle Powder

Humanity has always made an effort to maintain physical health and vigor throughout recorded history. People have looked for ways to retain good health and assume the physical forms they have always desired, whether in ancient civilizations or contemporary society. During this search, the "miracle powder" is discovered to be an intriguing and mysterious herbal cure that has captivated the interest of people all over the world. This chapter explores the origins, background, and cultural importance of the miracle powder, illuminating its traditional use and opening the door to its more recent usage in the field of belly fat reduction and natural weight loss.

Historical Significance and Origins

The locations where herbal knowledge flourished and indigenous wisdom was passed down through the generations are where the origins of the miracle powder can be found. Ancient cultures, including those in China, India, and Egypt, had great regard for the ability of plants and herbs to promote health and treat a range of illnesses. Blending powerful plant components together, the miracle powder became a treasured trade secret among shamans, herbalists, and healers.

The miracle powder's capacity to balance internal systems and harmonize the body's energy, or "qi," was acknowledged in ancient Chinese medicine. In a similar vein, Indian Ayurvedic doctors adopted the miracle powder into their comprehensive system of holistic health care, viewing it as a regulator of metabolism and intestinal health. The reputation of the miracle powder as a natural medicine with significant benefits on the human body was established by these old systems.

Ritualistic Traditions and Cultural Significance

In addition to its medicinal uses, the miracle powder had cultural value in many different communities. This herbal blend was prepared and consumed as part of ritualistic rites and practices. These customs helped people stay physically well while also strengthening their ties to their spiritual and cultural heritage.

The miracle powder was thought to have mystical abilities in certain civilizations, including the ability to call blessings or repel evil energies. Its inclusion in festivals, holy ceremonies, and rites of passage cemented its status as a representation of vigor and rebirth. The miracle powder was consumed in a reverent manner that encouraged a closer bond between the user and the natural environment.

Classic Applications and Hints

Beyond just helping people lose weight, the miracle powder was traditionally used for a host of other health benefits. It was acknowledged for its ability to boost immunity, ease gastrointestinal distress, and improve general vitality. Traditional healers and herbalists were aware of the complex interactions that exist between the human body and the botanical chemicals found in the miracle powder.

These practitioners created concoctions that utilized the synergy of various herbs, each of which contributed distinct properties to the mixture, by drawing on the knowledge of their forefathers. Carefully blended herbs, spices, and roots produced a holistic treatment that addressed the complex aspects of health. This comprehensive method supported the idea that genuine health results from a state of harmonious equilibrium encompassing the body, mind, and spirit.

Modern Resurrection and Modern Uses

There was a risk that conventional knowledge might become obsolete as the globe entered the contemporary era. But the charm of the magic powder remained, and its latest resurgence has been characterized by the fusion of traditional knowledge with cutting-edge research. The bioactive chemicals found in the miracle powder are being uncovered by researchers and health enthusiasts, providing insight into its possible advantages and modes of action.

The popularity of the miracle powder has returned due to the increased interest in holistic wellbeing, natural therapies, and sustainable weight management in today's society. Scientific studies into its effectiveness have been spurred by its well-established reputation as a herbal cure for reducing belly fat and weight loss. According to preliminary research, the miracle powder's botanical ingredients may affect metabolic pathways and encourage fat oxidation, which is consistent with its traditional use as a supplement to increase metabolism.

Through the pages of this book, we will travel back in time to discover the history of the miracle powder and explore its potential for natural weight loss. By establishing a connection between traditional wisdom and contemporary research, we can access a wealth of information that enables people to fully utilize the healing potential of this herbal treatment.

We set out on a journey of exploration, inspired by the need for holistic well-being in the present day and led by the wisdom of generations past, drawn by its fascinating past and promising future. The first chapter of the voyage delves into the history and cultural background of the miracle powder, providing a backdrop of insights that set the tone for the other chapters.

CHAPTER 2

Understanding Weight Loss and Belly Fat: Provide readers with a comprehensive overview of the science behind weight loss and the factors contributing to belly fat accumulation. Explain how the miracle powder's compounds interact with the body's metabolism.

The pursuit of weight loss has taken center stage in the lives of many people in the modern world. Diets, workout routines, and a wide range of weight reduction products have proliferated due to the desire to lose excess weight and obtain a healthier, thinner figure. The abdominal area is one of the most obstinate and worrisome places of fat growth. Not only does belly fat detract from one's appearance, but it is also associated with a number of health hazards, such as diabetes, metabolic disorders, and cardiovascular diseases. Understanding the complex mechanisms behind the buildup of belly fat and the underlying science guiding weight loss is essential for anyone starting a weight loss journey that will be effective. This chapter also explores possible interactions between the substances in the "miracle powder" and the metabolism of the body.

The Complete Guide to the Science of Weight Loss

The idea of energy balance is the foundation of weight loss. You have to burn more calories than you take in if you want to lose weight. Because of this imbalance, the body uses its fat reserves as fuel, which lowers the amount of fat in the body as a whole. The pace at which calories are expended is determined by the metabolic rate, which is regulated by a number of factors including age, gender, heredity, and degree of exercise. A balanced diet and regular exercise are essential for both achieving and maintaining weight loss. A calorie deficit is produced when one consumes less calories while exercising more, which promotes fat reduction.

Fat Belly: The Unwilling Build-Up

Visceral fat, or belly fat, is not the same as subcutaneous fat, which is located directly beneath the skin. Visceral fat is deposited around important organs such as the pancreas, liver, and intestines in the abdominal cavity. This ingrained fat has drawn notice because it is linked to health hazards that go beyond appearance. According to research, visceral fat is metabolically active and can release hormones and inflammatory chemicals that lead to insulin resistance, which is a risk factor for type 2 diabetes. Furthermore, metabolic problems and cardiovascular illnesses are directly associated with excess visceral fat.

Belly fat accumulates due to a number of circumstances. Where the body stores fat can be influenced by genetics. Abdominal fat storage may be exacerbated by hormones, especially the stress hormone cortisol. Poor eating habits, such as consuming a lot of processed and sugary foods, and sedentary lifestyles all lead to weight gain, particularly around the abdomen. Chronic stress and sleep deprivation might worsen the buildup of abdominal fat.

Interpreting the "Miracle Powder" and How It Affects Metabolism

For many people looking for quick fixes, the idea of a "miracle powder" that helps with weight loss has captivated their attention. A significant body of research is being done to determine the possible effects of specific chemicals on metabolism and fat reduction, even though such claims should be treated with care.

The substances in the miracle powder and the body's metabolism have intricate and varied relationships. A crucial element that is frequently emphasized is thermogenesis. The process by which the body produces heat and expels calories is known as thermogenesis. It has been demonstrated that some substances, like coffee and capsaicin from chili peppers, enhance thermogenesis.

Certain substances have the ability to trigger the production of hormones such as adrenaline, which can elevate heart rate and increase energy expenditure.

The control of appetite is an additional area of attention. Certain ingredients in the magic powder may affect hormones that regulate feelings of fullness and appetite, which could result in consuming fewer calories. For example, foods high in fiber might increase feelings of fullness, which can stop overeating.

Moreover, the magic powder may contribute to the oxidation of fat. The ability of substances like green tea extract to accelerate fat oxidation and increase the availability of stored fat for energy production has been researched. This may aid in the reduction of body fat overall, including abdominal fat.

It is imperative to stress, though, that a balanced diet and consistent exercise are the cornerstones of weight loss, and that no one powder or substance can take their place. Genetics, metabolism, and other factors can cause a large variation in an individual's body's reaction to these chemicals. Additionally, thorough scientific research is needed to determine the long-term safety and efficacy of such products.

Finitude

Making educated judgments about how to approach one's weight reduction journey requires an understanding of the science behind abdominal fat and weight loss. Because of the special way that fat accumulates in the belly area and the health problems that go along with it, it's critical to take a comprehensive approach that include healthy eating, exercise, stress reduction, and enough sleep. Although the idea of a "miracle powder" seems appealing, it's important to evaluate such claims cautiously and speak with medical experts before adding any new supplements to one's regimen. Ultimately, a combination of science, dedication, and customized tactics is required to achieve long-lasting weight loss and a healthier physique.

CHAPTER 3

The Science Behind the Miracle Powder: Delve into the biochemical and physiological mechanisms by which the miracle powder aids in weight loss and reduces belly fat. Explain how it impacts digestion, energy expenditure, and fat metabolism.

Finding the junction of current science and conventional knowledge can frequently provide remarkable insights in the quest for sustainable and effective weight loss. One prominent example of this confluence is the mysterious "miracle powder," which is praised for its ability to promote natural weight loss and decrease abdominal fat. This chapter delves deeply into the complex physiological and biochemical pathways that the miracle powder uses to work, providing insight into how it affects energy expenditure, fat metabolism, and digestion.

Metabolic Elegance and Digestive Harmony

The secret to the miracle powder's effectiveness is its capacity to balance the body's complex dance of digestion. Ancient societies understood that a healthy digestive system was essential to obtaining optimum health, and the miracle powder played a significant role in this story. Current research indicates that the blend of botanical chemicals in the miracle powder affects different phases of digestion, resulting in improvements to metabolism that help with weight loss.

The wonder powder promotes enzymatic activity, which is one of the main ways it aids with digestion. Some of the blend's herbs have been demonstrated to increase the production of digestive enzymes, which help to break down nutrients and make them easier to absorb and use. This series of enzyme activities guarantees effective digestion and keeps undigested materials from building up, which can lead to weight gain.

Additionally, the special blend of soluble and insoluble fibers in the miracle powder functions as a mild regulator of the digestive process. In the digestive system, soluble fibers congeal into a gel-like material that slows down nutrient absorption and increases feelings of fullness. Contrarily, insoluble fibers encourage frequent bowel motions and give stool more volume, which helps avoid the retention of waste that could impede weight loss attempts.

Thermogenesis and Energy Expenditure

The magic powder has an impact on more than just digestion—it also affects the complex domain of energy expenditure. The equilibrium between energy intake and energy expenditure is essential to the weight loss idea. The magic powder helps maintain this equilibrium by promoting thermogenesis, the body's mechanism of producing heat and burning energy.

It has been demonstrated that a few of the components in the miracle powder cause thermogenic pathways to fire. The process of thermogenesis increases calorie expenditure by converting fat, which is stored energy, into heat. This procedure helps reduce adipose tissue, especially in the abdominal area, in addition to aiding in weight loss.

Furthermore, the effects of the miracle powder on energy expenditure are not just immediate. Research indicates that it might contribute to increasing resting-state energy expenditure, or basal metabolic rate (BMR). Even when you're not exercising, your body burns more calories throughout the day when your BMR is greater. This helps you lose weight.

Lipid Oxidation and Fat Metabolism

The impact of the miracle powder on fat metabolism and lipid oxidation is among the most fascinating features of its process. One of the most critical aspects of losing weight and abdominal fat is effectively breaking down and using the fat that has been deposited. The components of the miracle powder have been shown to interact with lipid metabolism-related cellular receptors and enzymes, facilitating the conversion of triglycerides into fatty acids.

Its ability to increase lipid oxidation is another way that the miracle powder complements this lipolysis process. The magic powder leads to a decrease in fat storage, especially around the abdomen, by boosting the body's ability to burn fat for energy. This two-pronged strategy, which speeds up fat breakdown and encourages fat usage, highlights how comprehensive the miracle powder's weight loss benefits are.

The miracle powder plays a balancing role in the biochemistry and physiology symphony, directing a sequence of events that lead to a significant reduction in belly fat and weight loss. Its involvement in energy expenditure, fat metabolism, and digestion highlights its holistic approach to well-being, which is consistent with the holistic paradigms of traditional herbal medicine.

We have a greater understanding of the miracle powder's potential as a natural weight loss solution as we go through the complex network of pathways that underlie its effects. The fusion of traditional knowledge with modern research offers a fascinating picture of a herbal combination that supports the body's natural functions while also honoring them in the quest for overall well-being. Following the symphony of biochemical interactions that characterize the miracle powder's astonishing efficacy, we will continue to examine the transforming trip that it offers in the upcoming chapters.

CHAPTER 4

Choosing the Right Miracle Powder: Educate readers on the various types of miracle powders available, their sources, and preparation methods. Discuss the importance of quality, potency, and safety when selecting the right product.

Numerous solutions on the market promise speedy and revolutionary outcomes for those pursuing wellness and weight loss. These include the so-called "miracle powders," which are frequently promoted as effective tools for reaching fitness and health objectives. However, since not all miracle pills are made equal, traversing this terrain calls some discernment. This chapter explores the various kinds of miracle powders that are out there, their origins, methods of production, and how crucial it is to consider quality, potency, and safety when choosing the proper product.

A Range of Miracle Powders and Where to Find Them

Many different components can be found in miracle powders, and each one purports to have special advantages. Among the most prevalent kinds are:

1. Green Tea Extract: Made from Camellia sinensis leaves, green tea extract has chemicals including

catechins and antioxidants that are thought to help with fat oxidation and metabolism.

Turmeric Powder: Originating from the roots of the Curcuma longa plant, this bright yellow spice includes curcumin, which is well-known for its anti-inflammatory and maybe weight-management qualities.

The bark of Cinnamomum trees is the source of Cinnamon Powder, which is high in antioxidants and has been linked to better insulin sensitivity and metabolism control.

4. Garcinia Cambogia: This powder, which comes from a tropical fruit, is known to have the appetite-suppressing property of hydroxycitric acid (HCA).

5. Psyllium Husk Powder: This plant-based soluble fiber, which comes from the Plantago ovata plant, can support gut health, facilitate digestion, and encourage feelings of fullness.

Chia Seed Powder: Made from the seeds of the Salvia hispanica plant, this powder is rich in fiber and omega-3 fatty acids, which promote general health and satiety.

7. Moringa Powder: This powder is made from powdered Moringa oleifera leaves and is high in nutrients and antioxidants, which may help with metabolism and general well-being.

How to Prepare and How Much

Miracle powders are easy to incorporate into everyday routines because they may be used in a wide range of culinary creations and beverages. They can be used as a flavoring in cooking or added to smoothies, yogurt, and porridge. Some people choose to blend them into drinks by adding water or other liquids.

It's crucial to adhere to suggested dosage recommendations when utilizing these powders. Overindulgence could result in unexpected adverse consequences or drug interactions. As your body adjusts, it is best to gradually raise the dose from the lower starting point.

The Essential Elements: Safety, Potency, and Quality

It's important to prioritize quality, efficacy, and safety while choosing the best miracle powder rather than just going with the newest product. This is the reason these elements are crucial:

1. Quality: The miracle powder's quality is greatly influenced by the origin and manufacturing methods of its constituents. Organic and non-GMO sources are generally favored due to their reduced exposure to hazardous chemicals

and pesticides. Seek for goods from respectable companies that follow stringent quality assurance guidelines and independent testing.

2. Potency: A miracle powder's potency determines how effective it is. Active ingredients, like the catechins in green tea and the curcumin in turmeric, should be present in amounts that have been proved by science to have positive health effects. For details on the concentration of these active substances, consult the label.

3. Safety: There is no bargaining on safety. Speak with a healthcare provider before adding any new supplements, including magic powders, to your regimen. Certain substances may have negative effects on specific medical conditions or interact negatively with drugs. If you already take different supplements, take into account the combined effects.

4. Research and Reviews: Examine scholarly publications as well as user feedback. Look for research backing up the benefits that the particular magic powder you're

considering claims to offer. Genuine client testimonials can shed light on actual experiences and results.

5. Transparent Labeling: A reliable product will have labels that are easy to read and include a complete description of components, suppliers, and concentrations. Steer clear of products that make too dramatic or ambiguous claims.

6. Sustainable Sourcing : Take into account how the ingredients will affect the environment. Select

brands that place a high value on ethical and sustainable sourcing.

7. Long-Term Viability: Remember that although miracle powders may help in the short term, long-term weight loss and good health necessitate significant lifestyle adjustments. Products that guarantee miraculous transformations or overnight outcomes should be avoided.

Finitude

The effectiveness of miracle powders in assisting with health and weight loss objectives depends on a number of variables, including quality, potency, and safety. With so many different kinds of miracle powders on the market, people can customize their approach to suit their own tastes and requirements. These items should, though, be incorporated into a comprehensive health plan that also consists of a healthy diet, consistent exercise, stress reduction, and enough sleep. Making a point of putting trustworthy companies first, speaking with medical experts, and approaching these items critically can all assist people in making wise choices and reaping the rewards while preserving their health.

CHAPTER 5

Incorporating Miracle Powder into Your Diet: Provide practical tips and recipes for incorporating the miracle powder into daily meals and beverages. Highlight its versatility and compatibility with different cuisines.

The quest for natural weight loss and the decrease of abdominal fat is a dynamic investigation of balance and nutrition. The "miracle powder" must be seamlessly included into your regular food regimen in order for this quest to succeed. This chapter takes us on a culinary journey where we learn all the different ways that the miracle powder can be added to a wide range of dishes and drinks. It's a useful ally in your pursuit of holistic wellbeing because of its adaptability and compatibility with many types of food.

Welcoming Culinary Originality

With its diverse range of herbal ingredients, the miracle powder serves as a blank canvas that may be painted with an array of flavors and textures. Embracing culinary inventiveness is the first step towards introducing the miracle powder into your diet. Allow your creativity to go wild as you incorporate the essence of this herbal combination into your recipes for breakfast, supper, and every meal in between.

Morning Vitality: Breakfasts Packed with Power

Breakfast selections that are high in nutrients and use the magic powder will help you revitalize your mornings. Pour yourself a bowl of yogurt or porridge and top it with a dusting of the miracle powder to start your day. With this easy addition, your breakfast tastes even better and has the added benefit of increasing your metabolism. For a cool variation, mix the magic powder into a fruit smoothie to make a colorful drink that will invigorate your day.

World Fusion: Delightful Lunch and Dinner Options

Because the magic powder works with so many various kinds of food, you can experience a world of flavors. Add a pinch of the miracle powder and watch a simple salad become a flavor-filled treat. Stir it into stews, soups, and stir-fries to boost the nutritious value of your dishes and enjoy a subtle herbal flavor. Seamlessly blending into a tapestry of tastes, the miracle powder is perfect for meals with Mediterranean or Asian inspiration.

Drink and Taste: Herbal Concoctions and Drinks

Beyond meals, the miracle powder is a great fit for a range of calming, revitalizing, and energizing drinks. After steeping the magic powder in hot water, let the essence of the herbs slowly release into each drink to create a soothing herbal infusion. Blend it with freshly squeezed citrus juices for a zesty twist that will infuse your drink with a rush of herbal deliciousness. Transform a boring need into a restorative ritual by mixing the miracle powder into your water to enhance your hydration regimen.

Delicious Temptations: Nutritious Treats

Indulge your sweet taste without letting your dedication to natural weight loss slip. Discover the world of healthful goodies by adding the miracle powder to your baked goods, smoothie bowls, and homemade energy bars. Its delicate overtones bring out the natural sweetness of the ingredients, providing a guilt-free treat that advances your wellness goals.

A Bit of Guidance: Useful Recipes

In order to spark your creative juices, the following useful recipes highlight the many uses of the miracle powder:

1. A Morning Smoothie Miracle:

- Ingredients: Miracle powder, banana, chia seeds, spinach, Greek yogurt, and almond milk.

Directions: Process all ingredients in a blender until smooth. Apply a small amount of magic powder as a garnish.

2. Infusion of Herbal Herbs:

- Ingredients: Miracle powder, lemon juice, honey, and hot water.

The recipe calls for combining honey, lemon juice, and a small amount of miracle powder with hot water. Good stir, and savor.

3. Boost Your Mediterranean Salad:

- Ingredients: Miracle Powder Vinaigrette, feta cheese, olives, tomatoes, red onions, cucumbers, and mixed greens.

- Guidelines: Mix olive oil, lemon juice, miracle powder, and a small amount of honey with a whisk. Over the salad, drizzle, and toss.

4. A Stir-Fry Blended with Spice:

- Ingredients: Sesame oil, ginger, garlic, soy sauce, tofu or lean protein, and miracle powder.

Directions: Saute the protein and veggies, then mix in the soy sauce, sesame oil, ginger, garlic, and a dash of miracle powder to make a sauce.

5. Herbal Hydration Supplement:

Cold water, cucumber slices, mint leaves, lemon slices, and miracle powder are the ingredients.

- Directions: Put all the ingredients in a pitcher, cover, and refrigerate to steep. Present cold.

A Wholesome Gastronomic Adventure

Adding the magic powder to your diet is not just about making your food taste better; it's about discovering the harmonious relationship between the abundance of nature and your health. By infusing your food with the essence of this herbal blend, you are taking your palate on a holistic culinary adventure that honors the balance between flavor and nutrition. Because of the miracle powder's versatility in cooking, you can combine flavors to create a symphony that will not only tempt your palate but also help you achieve your objectives of losing belly fat and losing weight naturally. Now, spread open your culinary canvas and allow the magic powder to create a wellness masterpiece on your dish.

CHAPTER 6

Clinical Studies and Efficacy: Present an evidence-based chapter showcasing relevant scientific studies, clinical trials, and real-life success stories that support the miracle powder's effectiveness in promoting weight loss and reducing belly fat.

In a world full of claims of miraculous cures and cutting-edge technologies, astute buyers look for answers that are supported by data and can withstand close examination. This chapter explores clinical trials, real-world success stories, and scientific studies that support the miracle powder's efficacy in boosting weight loss and decreasing belly fat.

The Significance of Scientific Data

Credibility is based on scientific study, which distinguishes verified results from unsupported assertions. Thorough clinical research and trials shed light on the ways in which particular ingredients in the miracle powder interact with the body's metabolism to affect weight loss and reduce the amount of fat around the belly.

1. Green Tea Extract and Metabolism: A number of research works have looked into how green

tea extract affects how much weight is managed. Green tea's potent antioxidants, called catechins, have been demonstrated to improve fat oxidation and thermogenesis. Consuming green tea extract increased energy expenditure and fat oxidation, which may help reduce belly fat and total fat loss, according to a study published in the American Journal of Clinical Nutrition.

2. Curcumin and Inflammation: The anti-inflammatory qualities and possible metabolic consequences of the curcumin

component in turmeric have drawn interest. Participants in a randomized controlled research showed that taking curcumin supplements significantly reduced their waist circumference and body weight. The trial was published in the Journal of Nutritional Science and Vitaminology.

3. Dietary Fiber and fullness: It is commonly known that dietary fiber helps to promote fullness and aid in weight management. An investigation of the effects of psyllium husk supplementation on body composition was conducted

and published in the Journal of the American College of Nutrition. Increased sensations of fullness and decreased calorie intake were observed in psyllium-consuming participants, indicating a potential role for fiber-rich miracle powders in weight loss.

4. Actual Success Stories in Life: Although clinical research offers significant insights, an approachable aspect of miracle powders' effectiveness is provided by real-life success tales. Many people have written testimonials and posted their experiences online,

crediting the use of these powders in their regimens for their weight loss and reduction of belly fat. But it's important to approach these kinds of stories with critical eyes, understanding that people may react differently from one another.

Moving Through the Evidence Landscape

Even if these research and success stories offer encouraging hints about the possible advantages of miracle powders, it's crucial to consider the information in light of a larger body of scientific knowledge. Results can be influenced by variables like doses, individual variability, and study methods.

1. Studies' Quality: Evaluate the studies' quality. When determining causality and generalizability, bigger sample numbers and randomized controlled studies with placebo groups are more reliable.

2. Consistency: Examine results for consistency across several investigations. Results that are repeated support the veracity of statements.

3. Dosage and Duration : Take into account the research-derived dosages and durations. You can increase the probability that you will reap similar advantages from miracle powders by simulating these settings when using them.

4. Individual Factors: Remember that a person's response may differ depending on their history, metabolism, way of living, and general state of health.

5. Holistic Approach: Although miracle powders can help with

weight loss, keep in mind that a balanced diet, consistent exercise, and good lifestyle choices are necessary for long-term success.

Finitude

Clinical research, clinical trials, and real-world success stories come together to offer a comprehensive view of the effectiveness of miracle powders in encouraging weight reduction and decreasing visceral fat. These data-driven observations provide a starting point for anyone looking for scientifically validated ways to improve their journey toward wellbeing. It's crucial to have a critical mindset, speak with medical professionals, and incorporate miracle powders into a holistic plan for long-term fitness and health goals when investigating these options.

CHAPTER 7

Combining Herbal Remedies and Lifestyle Changes: Offer holistic strategies for achieving sustainable weight loss by combining the use of the miracle powder with other herbal remedies, exercise routines, and mindful eating habits.

The road to success in the quest for long-term weight loss and overall wellbeing is not laid by a single answer, but rather by the skillful blending of numerous components that assist your path. This chapter offers a step-by-step plan for using the potency of the "miracle powder" in conjunction with intentional exercise regimens, mindful eating practices, and supplementary herbal medicines to help you achieve your wellness goals. You'll set out on a transformative journey toward a healthier, more vibrant you by adopting these holistic tactics.

The symbiotic dance: the miracle powder and herbal remedies

Even if the miracle powder is the star of the show, it's important to recognize the power of synergy that arises when it joins forces with other herbal companions. Adding herbs that are recognized for improving digestion, promoting metabolism, or reducing stress can enhance the efficacy of the miracle powder. For example, combining the miracle powder with green tea, which is well known for its thermogenic properties, results in a potent combination that increases energy expenditure and fat burning.

You can deliberately mix herbal tinctures, infusions, or pills to build a personalized regimen that supports your unique wellness objectives. Speak with a healthcare provider or herbalist before starting any herbal journey to make sure your plan is customized to meet your specific needs and maximize safety and effectiveness.

Starting an Odyssey of Movement: Intentional Exercise

Engaging in physical activity is a fundamental component of a comprehensive weight loss regimen. The ability of the miracle powder to increase energy expenditure and encourage fat metabolism is best suited for an organized workout program. Regularly performing aerobic workouts, weight training, and flexibility-building exercises increases your resting metabolic rate while burning calories and building lean muscle mass.

Think about creating a customized fitness regimen that fits your tastes and way of life. Include enjoyable activities in your routine, like cycling, yoga, dance, or brisk walks, to maintain consistency and long-term growth. Exercise fuels your body's energy expenditure while the miracle powder supports your metabolism, resulting in a synergistic cycle of transformation.

Contemplative Eating: A Fulfilling Tradition

In today's world of hectic schedules and diversions, eating frequently turns into a mindless ritual. On the other hand, mindful eating promotes a significant shift in awareness by encouraging you to appreciate each bite, pay attention to your body's signals, and develop a closer relationship with the food you eat. Using the miracle powder in conjunction with mindful eating techniques increases the effectiveness of your weight loss efforts.

Start by setting up a calm, distraction-free dining area. Take a minute to be grateful for the food that is in front of you as you settle down to eat it, laced with the magic powder. Use all of your senses to appreciate every taste, texture, and scent. Pay attention to your body's signals of hunger and fullness, and let it make the natural decisions about how much food to eat.

Creating Your Personalized Holistic Plan

To incorporate the miracle powder into your overall health regimen, several components must be carefully coordinated. This is a road map to help you along the way:

First, Herbal Symphony : Look into and choose supplementary herbal treatments that support your objectives. To fully utilize the potential of the miracle powder, create a safe and efficient herbal regimen by consulting a professional.

2. Energizing Movement: Create a workout plan that incorporates strength training, flexibility exercises, and cardiovascular activities. Make the program fit your needs and stick to a regular schedule to keep the momentum going.

3. Mindful Mastery: Develop a closer relationship with your meals and establish a calm dining space as you embrace mindful eating techniques. Taste the flavors of recipes made with miracle powder while paying attention to your body's signals.

4. Consistency and Patience : Recognize that change happens gradually. Accept consistency in your mindful eating, workout regimen, and herbal medicines. Have patience with yourself and

acknowledge your little accomplishments as you go.

5. Holistic Support: Consult medical doctors, herbalists, exercise specialists, and wellness groups for advice and support. Be in the company of people who are as dedicated to holistic well-being as you are.

Your Holistic Transformation Unveiled

Through the integration of the miracle powder with intentional movement, mindful nutrition, and supplementary herbal medicines, you can experience a comprehensive change that goes beyond weight reduction. The combination of these components supports not just your physical health but also your mental, emotional, and spiritual well. Remember that every step you take on this life-changing journey is an indication of your commitment to holistic wellness and your acceptance of a life that is harmonious, balanced, and full of vitality.

CHAPTER 8

Precautions and Considerations: Address potential side effects, contraindications, and interactions of the miracle powder with medications or existing health conditions. Provide guidance on proper dosages and the importance of consulting a healthcare professional.

It's critical to approach dietary supplements with a clear knowledge of potential hazards and interactions when people set out on journeys towards better health and weight management. This chapter delves further into the important subject of safety measures and things to think about when utilizing miracle powders. Comprehending these elements is crucial for safe and efficient use, as they include potential adverse effects, contraindications, and interactions with medications or medical conditions.

1. Possible Adverse Reactions

Even while miracle powders are frequently made from natural ingredients, they can sometimes have negative consequences, particularly if taken in excess or by people who have certain sensitivity issues. Allergic responses, gastric distress, and drug interactions are examples of common adverse effects. It's critical to keep an eye on your body's reaction and to stop using the product if negative consequences occur.

2.   Contraindications and Medication Interactions

Certain ingredients in miracle powders have the potential to worsen pre-existing medical issues or interfere with drugs. For example:

- Blood Thinners: The blood-thinning qualities of turmeric and green tea extract may interact with anticoagulant drugs, increasing the risk of bleeding.

Medications for Diabetes: Certain magic powders, like cinnamon, have the ability to decrease blood sugar. People who take diabetic medication need to be cautious in order to avoid hypoglycemia.

Diseases of the Gastrointestines: High-fiber wonder powders may make diseases of the gastrointestinal tract worse, such as inflammatory bowel disease (IBD) and irritable bowel syndrome (IBS).

Allergies: Miracle powders made from certain plants or compounds should be used with caution by people who are allergic to those substances.

3. Medical Professional Consultation and Dosage

A miracle powder's recommended dosage must be carefully calculated taking into account variables like age, weight, health, and the concentration of the particular ingredient. It's critical to abide by dose recommendations made by medical specialists or found on product labels. It can be helpful to start with a lesser dose and increase it gradually to see how your body reacts.

4. Breastfeeding and Pregnancy

Miracle powder users who are expecting or nursing should use caution when using these products because some of the chemicals could be harmful to the growing fetus or baby. During this time, it is imperative that you speak with a healthcare professional before starting any new supplement regimen.

5. Health Issues That Were Present Before

Before utilizing miracle powders, anyone with pre-existing medical illnesses, such as kidney, liver, or cardiovascular ailments, should speak with a healthcare provider. Certain substances may interfere with drugs provided for various illnesses or alter how well organs operate.

6. All-Inclusive Method

It is not appropriate to think about miracle powders as stand-alone fixes. Although they may help with weight management and general health, a holistic approach is the most effective way to fully reap their benefits. The cornerstones of a successful and long-lasting wellness journey include stress management, a balanced diet, consistent exercise, and enough sleep.

7. Speaking with health care providers

Above all, before adding magic powders to your regimen, it is imperative that you speak with healthcare specialists. This is especially true if you have pre-existing medical conditions, are taking medication, or are expecting or nursing a child. Healthcare professionals are able to provide individualized advice based on your unique needs and medical history.

Finitude

Miracle powders show potential as supplements that could help achieve health and weight-loss objectives. To reduce any dangers, however, informed and cautious use is crucial. People can make educated selections if they are aware of possible side effects, drug interactions, and contraindications. It is crucial to speak with medical professionals since their knowledge guarantees that using magic powders in accordance with your demands will maximize benefits and minimize hazards.